Annals of the ICRP

ICRP PUBLICATION 132

Radiological Protection from Cosmic Radiation in Aviation

Editor-in-Chief
C.H. CLEMENT

Associate Editor
N. HAMADA

Authors on behalf of ICRP
J. Lochard, D.T. Bartlett, W. Rühm, H. Yasuda,
J-F. Bottollier-Depois

PUBLISHED FOR

The International Commission on Radiological Protection

by

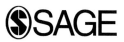

Please cite this issue as 'ICRP, 2016. Radiological protection
from cosmic radiation in aviation. ICRP Publication 132.
Ann. ICRP 45(1), 1–48.'

1

CONTENTS

EDITORIAL 5

ABSTRACT 9

PREFACE 11

MAIN POINTS 13

GLOSSARY 15

1. INTRODUCTION 21

    1.1. Background 21
    1.2. Scope 22
    1.3. Structure of the publication 22

2. CHARACTERISTICS OF EXPOSURE TO COSMIC RADIATION IN
   AVIATION 23

    2.1. Historical background 23
    2.2. Source and pathways 23
    2.3. Solar flares 25
    2.4. Assessment of individual exposure in aircraft 28
    2.5. Exposure of aircraft crew 29
    2.6. Epidemiological studies of aircraft crew 32

3. THE ICRP SYSTEM OF PROTECTION FOR PASSENGERS AND
   AIRCRAFT CREW 33

    3.1. Types of exposure situation and categories of exposure 33
    3.2. Justification of protection strategies 34
    3.3. Optimisation of protection 35

4. IMPLEMENTATION OF THE ICRP SYSTEM OF PROTECTION 37

    4.1. Protective actions 37
    4.2. Graded approach 38
    4.3. Protection of embryo and fetus 40
    4.4. Information dissemination to the general public and stakeholder
       engagement 41

5. CONCLUSIONS... 43

REFERENCES.. 45

ANNEX A. COSMIC RADIATION EXPOSURE ASSOCIATED WITH
SELECTED FLIGHT ROUTES... 48

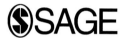

ICRP Publication 132

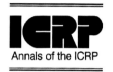

Editorial

TAKING FLIGHT IN A SEA OF COSMIC RADIATION

Ionising radiation is ubiquitous in the natural world. Thorium, uranium, and potassium – naturally radioactive elements created at the centre of the Sun, long before Earth was formed – and their decay products were here before there was life on Earth, and will still be here a billion years from now. They are found in varying degrees in rocks, soil, water, air, plants, animals, and humans. In addition to radiation from the earth, we are exposed to cosmic radiation from the Sun and outer space, generated in the chaotic formation of the universe and by the massive processes that fuel the stars. Life on earth evolved in this 'sea of radiation', and future generations will live in it just as we do now.

Ionising radiation cannot be sensed directly, and it was only upon the discovery of x rays in 1895 by Wilhelm Röntgen (Röntgen, 1895) that its existence became apparent. The following year, Henri Becquerel discovered that radiation is part of the natural environment (Becquerel, 1896a,b). Cosmic radiation was discovered 16 years later by Victor Hess in experiments involving high-altitude balloon flights (Hess, 1912).

For many decades, radiological protection focused on radiation sources made or concentrated by humans, such as x rays, and radioisotopes created in nuclear reactors and accelerators. However, certain natural sources, notably radon, started to receive more attention in recent decades. Exposure to radon represents half of the average worldwide dose from natural radiation (UNSCEAR, 2010). The International Commission on Radiological Protection (ICRP) addressed radiological protection related to radon exposure most recently in *Publication 126* (ICRP, 2014).

Daily exposure to cosmic radiation is also a natural part of the environment in which we live. Until recent decades, it was considered to be of minor relevance, as Earth's magnetic field and atmosphere provide protection from cosmic radiation. Now, however, over 500 astronauts have gone beyond this protection and faced significantly higher cosmic radiation dose rates, and this number will increase in the future. This specific circumstance was addressed in *Publication 123* entitled 'Assessment of radiation exposure of astronauts in space' (ICRP, 2013).

In addition, nowadays, given the increase in commercial air travel, exposure to cosmic radiation is also of importance for aircraft crew and passengers. When we travel at altitude, we are exposed to higher levels of cosmic radiation than at ground level. At typical commercial flight altitudes, the dose rate is generally in the range of $2-10\,\mu Sv\,h^{-1}$, depending primarily on latitude, altitude, and level of solar activity (ICRU, 2010). Hundreds of flying hours per year are needed for this dose to be significant compared with the annual dose due to other exposures from natural radiation, for which the worldwide average is 2400 μSv, and the typical range is 1000–13,000 μSv (UNSCEAR, 2010). As such, this publication focuses on aircraft crew and frequent flyers, some of whom spend many hundreds of hours in the air each year.

Cosmic radiation in the atmosphere occurs as both primary and secondary fields with complex particle composition and energy. Measurement of dose for aircraft crew and passengers is difficult, as instruments capable of monitoring the total field spectrum are generally bulky and not very robust. As a result, research over the past two decades has concentrated on dose assessment based on software programme codes. The use of codes is possible because the radiation field is relatively constant; changes in local area doses occur rarely and only in association with solar-generated ground-level enhancements. These codes rely on knowing aircraft latitudes, longitudes, and barometric altitudes on the routes flown, usually presented as a flight plan.

Internationally, there are more than 11 tested and proven codes or models that allow doses to aircraft crew and passengers to be determined with error margins within ±20% of the measured median. This is considered to be acceptable in scientific circles as the codes usually provide conservative estimates.

Since 1996, aircraft crew in the European Union have been recognised as occupationally exposed workers at typical flight altitudes of 8–12 km. As such, all European air carriers are required to keep records of aircraft crew exposure. Since 2006, compliance has been directed by EURATOM/96/29 (EURATOM, 2006), and has been implemented by all states. Similarly, in the 1990s, Canada adopted the recommendations in *Publication 60* (ICRP, 1991) and required radiation monitoring of aircraft crew, which led to the development of the PCAIRE programme. In 2006, the Japanese Radiation Council published guidelines for monitoring and management of doses to aircraft crew, and strongly urged national and domestic airlines to perform such record keeping voluntarily.

The USA promotes radiation safety of aircraft crew through educational materials on radiation exposure and recommended limits produced by the Federal Aviation Administration's Civil Aerospace Medical Institute. It has produced computer programmes that use the same flight planning parameters discussed above, and promotes self-monitoring and guidance for individual assessment of exposure and work regime, but does not mandate formal airline monitoring programmes.

These codes make the assessment of dose relatively straightforward, and this is a critical step in radiological protection. Subsequent steps involve the examination of protection options, and the optimisation of protection using individual dose criteria to avoid unacceptable exposure and inequity in dose distribution.

In *Publication 103* (ICRP, 2007), the Commission introduced three exposure situations: planned, existing, and emergency. These situations, along with the exposure categories (public, occupational, and medical), help clarify the most appropriate approach for radiological protection in any particular situation.

This publication affirms that exposure to cosmic radiation is an existing exposure situation, as the source exists before protection decisions can be made. In addition, this publication affirms that exposure of aircraft crew to cosmic radiation is occupational, and thus employers have a role to play in protection, even if options are limited in this case. There is no contradiction in this. Occupational exposures can occur in existing exposure situations, and this does not imply that protection measures cannot be planned.

The general approach of optimisation of protection with restrictions on individual dose applies in all circumstances. The exposure category and the type of exposure situation will influence how this is achieved. Furthermore, specific circumstances dictate which measures are practical, effective, and worthwhile. This publication provides radiological protection recommendations specific to cosmic radiation in aviation.

IAN GETLEY

CHRISTOPHER CLEMENT
ICRP SCIENTIFIC SECRETARY
EDITOR-IN-CHIEF

REFERENCES

Becquerel, H., 1896a. Sur les radiations émises par phosphorescence. Comptes Rendus 122, 420–421.

Becquerel, H., 1896b. Sur les radiations émises par phosphorescence. Comptes Rendus 122, 501–503.

EURATOM, 2006. Council Directive 96/29/Euratom of 13 May 1996 Laying Down Basic Safety Standards for the Protection of the Health of Workers and the General Public Against the Dangers Arising from Ionizing Radiation. Off. J. Eur. Commun. No L 159/1. Available at: http://eur-lex.europa.eu/legal-content/EN/TXT/PDF/?uri = CELEX:01996L0029-20000513&from = EN (last accessed 14 May 2016).

Hess, V.F., 1912. Über Beobachtungen der durchdringenden Strahlung bei sieben Freiballonfahrten. Physikalische Zeitschrift 13, 1084–1091.

ICRP, 1991. Recommendations of the International Commission on Radiological Protection. ICRP Publication 60. Ann. ICRP 21(1–3).

ICRP, 2007. The 2007 Recommendations of the International Commission on Radiological Protection. ICRP Publication 103. Ann. ICRP 37(2–4).

ICRP, 2013. Assessment of radiation exposure of astronauts in space. ICRP Publication 123. Ann. ICRP 42(4).

ICRP, 2014. Radiological protection against radon exposure. ICRP Publication 126. Ann. ICRP 43(3).

ICRU, 2010. Reference data for the validation of doses from cosmic-radiation exposure of aircraft crew. Report 84. J. ICRU 10(2).

Röntgen, W., 1895. Über eine neue Art von Strahlen. Sitzungsberichte der Würzburger Physik-medic. Gesellschaft 22, 153–157.

UNSCEAR, 2010. Sources and Effects of Ionizing Radiation. UNSCEAR 2008 Report to the General Assembly. United Nations Scientific Committee on the Effects of Atomic Radiation. United Nations, New York.

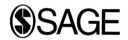
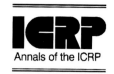

Annals of the ICRP

Radiological Protection from Cosmic Radiation in Aviation

ICRP PUBLICATION 132

Approved by the Commission in March 2016

Abstract–In this publication, the International Commission on Radiological Protection (ICRP) provides updated guidance on radiological protection from cosmic radiation in aviation, taking into account the current ICRP system of radiological protection, the latest available data on exposures in aviation, and experience gained worldwide in the management of exposures in aviation. The publication describes the origins of cosmic radiation, how it exposes passengers and aircraft crew, the basic radiological protection principles that apply to this existing exposure situation, and the available protective actions. For implementation of the optimisation principle, the Commission recommends a graded approach proportionate to the level of exposure that may be received by individuals. The objective is to keep the exposure of the most exposed individuals to a reasonable level. The Commission also recommends that information be disseminated to raise awareness about cosmic radiation, and to support informed decisions among concerned stakeholders.

Keywords: Cosmic radiation; Aviation; Aircraft crew; Frequent flyers; Graded approach

AUTHORS ON BEHALF OF ICRP
J. LOCHARD, D.T. BARTLETT, W. RÜHM,
H. YASUDA, J-F. BOTTOLLIER-DEPOIS

PREFACE

'Well, I made it!' were the first words of the aviator Charles Lindbergh after the *Spirit of St. Louis* touched down at Le Bourget airport after flying 5800 km from Long Island (The New York Times, 1924). The observers of the time emphasised the courage of the pioneer against the cold, the weather conditions, and the tiredness; no one talked about radiation exposure, and with good reason. Only a handful of scientists were aware of cosmic radiation at that time. This pioneering performance opened the way for transcontinental flights. Since Charles Lindbergh's flight, the increase in aircraft performance and capacity, low-cost companies, and expansion of tourism have led to large increases in the number of air passengers. In 2014, approximately 3.2 billion flight tickets were sold, and this figure is expected to double by 2030 (ICAO, 2015). Furthermore, the business jet market continues to grow at approximately 4% per year, and the fleet is expected to double by 2032. This raises the potential for a significant increase in individual and collective exposure of aircraft crew and passengers to cosmic radiation.

In this context, at a meeting in Cape Town, South Africa, in October 2010, the Main Commission of the International Commission on Radiological Protection (ICRP) approved the formation of Task Group 83, reporting to Committee 4, to develop guidance on radiological protection against exposure to cosmic radiation in aviation.

The terms of reference of Task Group 83 were to prepare a report that describes and clarifies the application of the 2007 Recommendations (ICRP, 2007) for the protection of aircraft crew and passengers, particularly frequent flyers, against exposure to cosmic radiation. The report should discuss the type of exposure situation relevant to the control of exposures in aviation, and the appropriate radiological protection principles to be implemented. Particular attention should be given to implementation of the optimisation principle, which is the cornerstone of the system of radiological protection recommended by the Commission.

The membership of Task Group 83 was as follows:

J. Lochard (Chair)	J-F. Bottollier-Depois	W. Rühm
D.T. Bartlett	R. Hunter	H. Yasuda

The corresponding member was:

S. Mundigl

Committee 4 critical reviewers were:

D.A. Cool	M. Kai

Main Commission critical reviewers were:

H. Liu   S. Romanov

Sylvain Andresz played an important role in development of this report, providing welcome scientific and editorial assistance. Numerous helpful comments were also received from Gerhard Frasch, Gérard Desmaris, and Frank Bonnotte. The Task Group would like to thank them all, as well as Le Centre d'étude sur l'Evaluation de la Protection dans le domaine Nucléaire (CEPN), for their valuable support.

Task Group 83 met on 1–2 February 2011 at the premises of CEPN at Fontenay-aux-Roses, France, and then worked by correspondence.

The membership of Committee 4 during the period of preparation of this report was:

(2009–2013)

J. Lochard (Chair)	T. Homma	G. Massera
W. Weiss (Vice-Chair)	M. Kai	K. Mrabit
J-F. Lecomte (Secretary)	H. Liu	S. Shinkarev
P. Burns	S. Liu	J. Simmonds
P. Carboneras	A. McGarry	A. Tsela
D.A. Cool	S. Magnusson	W. Zeller

(2013–2017)

D.A. Cool (Chair)	M. Doruff	A. Nisbet
K-W. Cho (Vice-Chair)	E. Gallego	D. Oughton
J-F. Lecomte (Secretary)	T. Homma	T. Pather
F. Bochud	M. Kai	S. Shinkarev
M. Boyd	S. Liu	J. Takala
A. Canoba	A. McGarry	

MAIN POINTS

- Cosmic radiation is composed of high-energy particles originating from space and from the Sun. Basically, the higher the altitude and the latitude, the higher the dose rate. A rapid increase in dose rate can occur in connection with solar flares. As a result, flying in aircraft increases exposure to cosmic radiation.
- Considering that the number of passengers will continue to increase, and aircraft technology will enable aircraft to fly for longer durations and at higher altitudes, cumulative exposures of aircraft crew and passengers to cosmic radiation are likely to increase. The Commission therefore considers that it is important to develop and implement a protection strategy.
- The Commission considers exposure to cosmic radiation, including that produced by solar flares, as an existing exposure situation.
- The Commission continues to consider that the exposure of all aircraft passengers, both occasional and frequent flyers for personal reasons or professional duties, should be regarded as public exposure, and that the exposure of aircraft crew should be treated as occupational exposure.
- The Commission recommends that exposure be maintained as low as reasonably achievable with a dose reference level selected to take into account the level of exposure of the most exposed individuals who warrant specific attention in the particular circumstance, typically in the 5–10 mSv year^{-1} range.
- For practical implementation of the protection strategy, the Commission recommends a graded approach based on the flight frequency of the individuals.
  - Most passengers in aircraft are occasional flyers, and their exposure to cosmic radiation is considered to be negligible in the context of their total radiation exposure. However, the Commission recommends that general information about cosmic radiation be made available to all passengers.
  - For frequent flyers for personal reasons or professional duties, in addition to the recommendation to provide general information, the Commission encourages self-assessment of doses to enable individuals to consider adjustment of their flight frequency if they feel the need.
  - For the small fraction of frequent flyers for professional duties whose exposures are comparable to those of aircraft crew, the Commission recommends that the requirements for such flyers be decided on a case-by-case basis through interactions between the individual and their organisation, according to the prevailing circumstances.
  - For aircraft crew, the Commission recommends that the operating management:
    - (i) inform the aircraft crew individually about cosmic radiation through an educational programme;
    - (ii) assess the dose of aircraft crew;
    - (iii) record the individual and cumulative dose of aircraft crew. These data should be made available to the individuals and should be kept for a reasonable period of time that is, at a minimum, comparable with the expected lifetime of the individuals; and

(iv) adjust the flight roster when appropriate, considering the selected dose reference level and after consultation with the concerned aircraft crew.

- For most purposes, use of one of the properly validated calculation programmes is considered sufficient for assessment of dose for aircraft crew and passengers.
- Pregnant frequent flyers for personal reasons or professional duties may wish to adjust their flight frequency to reduce the exposure of their embryo/fetus to cosmic radiation based on self-assessment of exposure. For pregnant aircraft crew, airline management should have provisions in place to adjust duties during the remainder of the pregnancy after its notification, consistent with the Commission's recommendations.
- The Commission also recommends that national authorities or airline companies disseminate information to raise awareness about cosmic radiation and support informed decisions among all concerned stakeholders, and foster a radiological protection culture for occupationally exposed individuals.

GLOSSARY[1]

Categories of exposure

The Commission distinguishes between three categories of radiation exposure: occupational, public, and medical.

Cosmic radiation

Cosmic radiation is ionising radiation that consists of high-energy particles, primarily atomic nuclei, of extraterrestrial origin, and particles generated by interaction with the atmosphere and other matter.

Primary cosmic radiation is cosmic radiation incident from space and the Sun at the Earth's orbit.

Secondary cosmic radiation comprises particles that are created directly or in a cascade of reactions by primary cosmic radiation interacting with the atmosphere or other matter. Important particles with respect to radiological protection and radiation measurement in aircraft are: neutrons, protons, photons, electrons, positrons, muons, and, to a lesser extent, pions and nuclear ions heavier than protons.

Galactic cosmic radiation is cosmic radiation that originates outside the solar system.

Solar cosmic radiation is cosmic radiation from the Sun.

Dose criteria

The generic designation of any criterion of individual dose established as part of a radiological protection programme for the purpose of providing a boundary for optimisation of protection, to address inequity, and to ensure adequate protection. The Commission's terms 'reference level', 'dose constraint', and 'dose limit' are all examples of dose criteria in particular circumstances.

Embryo

Unborn human in early stages of development in the uterus (before 3 months of gestation).

---

[1] At the time of issuance of this publication, the Commission was revising the glossary enclosed in *Publication 103* (ICRP, 2007) because of some imperfections and inconsistencies. Note that in this publication, definitions refer to those found in the text of *Publication 103* rather than its glossary.

Emergency exposure situation

Emergency exposure situations are exposure situations resulting from a loss of control of a planned source, or from any unexpected event involving an uncontrolled source (e.g. a malevolent event). These situations require urgent and timely actions in order to avoid or mitigate exposure.

Employer

An organisation, corporation, partnership, firm, association, trust, estate, public or private institution, group, political or administrative entity, or other persons designated in accordance with national legislation with recognised responsibility, commitment, and duties towards a worker in her or his employment by virtue of a mutually agreed relationship.

Existing exposure situations

Existing exposure situations are exposure situations resulting from sources that already exist when a decision to control the resulting exposure is taken. These include natural sources (cosmic radiation, radon, and other naturally occurring radioactive materials) and man-made sources (long-term exposure from past practices, accidents, or radiological events). Characterisation of exposures is a prerequisite to their control.

Exposure situation

A situation where a natural or man-made radiation source is transferred through various pathways, and the radiation results in exposure of humans or other biota.

Exposure pathway

A route by which radiation or radionuclides can reach humans and cause exposure.

Fetus

Unborn human in the uterus when fully developed (after 3 months of gestation).

Fluence

Fluence is the quotient of the number of particles incident upon a sphere of cross-sectional area. Fluence is measured in m^{-2}.

Frequent flyer

A person who travels regularly by aircraft, for personal reasons or professional duties, and who may be registered in a frequent flyer programme. Some frequent flyers may reach an annual flight time that is of the order of magnitude of typical aircraft crew (e.g. $500\,h\,year^{-1}$).

Ground-level enhancement

When solar flares emit cosmic rays of sufficient energy and intensity to raise radiation levels on Earth's surface to the degree that they are detected readily by neutron monitors, they are termed 'ground-level enhancements or events'.

Graded approach

A graded approach aims to ensure that the Commission's recommendations or requisites formulated for a group of individuals are commensurate and proportionate with their level of exposure, also considering the prevailing circumstances.

Justification

The process of determining whether: (i) a planned activity involving radiation is beneficial overall (i.e. whether the benefits to individuals and to society from introducing or continuing the activity outweigh the harm resulting from the activity); or (ii) the decision to control exposure in an emergency or existing exposure situation is likely to be beneficial overall (i.e. whether the benefits to individuals and society outweigh its cost and any harm or damage it causes).

Occasional flyer

A person who travels by air from time to time, reaching an annual flight time distinctly below that of typical aircraft crew.

Occupational exposure

Occupational exposure refers to all exposure of workers incurred as a result of their work; however, because of the ubiquity of radiation, the Commission limits its use of 'occupational exposure' to radiation exposures incurred at work as a result of situations that can reasonably be regarded as being the responsibility of the operating management.

Operating management

The person or group of persons that directs, controls, and assesses an organisation at the highest level. Many different terms are used, including chief executive officer, director general, managing director, and executive group.

Optimisation of protection

The principle of optimisation of radiological protection is a source-related process that aims to keep the magnitude of individual doses, the number of people exposed, and the likelihood of potential exposure as low as reasonably achievable below the appropriate dose criteria (constraint or reference level), economic and societal factors being taken into account.

Planned exposure situations

Planned exposure situations are exposure situations resulting from the deliberate introduction and operation of radiation sources. Planned exposure situations can be anticipated and fully controlled.

Principles of protection

Three basic principles structure the system of radiological protection: the principle of justification and the principle of optimisation of protection that apply to all controllable exposure situations, and the principle of application of dose limits that only applies to planned exposure situations.

Protective action

Action set to protect people from the harm of ionising radiation. Protective actions are generally those that influence the distance to the source, time of exposure, or shielding.

Reference level

In emergency and existing exposure situations, this dose criterion represents the level of dose or risk above which it is judged to be inappropriate to plan to allow exposures to occur, and below which optimisation of protection should be implemented. The chosen value for a reference level will depend upon the prevailing circumstances of the exposures under consideration.

Right to know

The principle according to which patients, workers, and members of the public have the right to be informed about what hazards they are exposed to and how to protect themselves, consistent with the ethical values of autonomy, justice, and prudence.

Risk

Risk relates to the probability that an outcome (e.g. cancer) will occur. Terms relating to risk are grouped together here:

Excess relative risk is the rate of disease in an exposed population divided by the rate of the disease in an unexposed population minus 1. This is often expressed as the excess relative risk per Sv.

Relative risk is the rate of disease in an exposed population divided by the rate of the disease in an unexposed population.

Solar flare

A solar flare is a large emission of energetic solar particles ejected into space by the Sun. The frequency of occurrence varies with solar activity from less than one per week to several per day. Large solar flares are less frequent than smaller solar flares. Solar flares can produce a stream of energetic particles in the solar wind known as 'solar proton events'. When these particles can be observed by ground-based cosmic radiation detectors, they are called 'ground-level events or enhancements'.

Solar wind

The solar wind is a plasma of electrons, protons, and alpha particles that boils off the solar corona and propagates – due to the Sun's magnetic field – radially from the Sun at an average velocity of $400\,\text{km s}^{-1}$. The solar wind carries with it a relatively strong and convoluted magnetic field that affects the fluence of galactic cosmic radiation. The solar wind is responsible for the aurora in the Arctic (*aurora borealis*) and the Antarctic (*aurora australis*).

1. INTRODUCTION

(1) Reaching one's seat in an aircraft can sometimes be a long journey. After check-in and passport control, one has to undergo airport security. Radiation may play a role in this process as it is used to screen carry-on luggage, and, in some cases, to screen individuals. The Commission has recently published recommendations on radiological protection for security screening (ICRP, 2014).

(2) After take-off, as the aircraft climbs to cruising altitude, exposure to cosmic radiation increases. At typical cruising altitude (>10,000 m), the dose rate can reach $7 \mu Sv h^{-1}$ (more than 150 times the level of exposure to cosmic radiation at sea level). Future use of new ultra-long-range jets that fly at higher altitudes and for longer durations is estimated to increase total doses by 30–50% compared with current flight practices [estimation by *Vereiningung Cockpit*, Germany and cited by Frasch et al. (2012)].

(3) Previously, the Commission developed a set of recommendations focusing specifically on the radiological protection of aircraft crew, paying particular attention to pregnant aircraft crew (ICRP, 1984, 1991). The present publication will review these recommendations, and also consider the exposure of passengers, particularly frequent flyers travelling for personal reasons or professional duties.

1.1. Background

(4) The Commission first mentioned exposure resulting from flying at high altitude in *Publication 9* (ICRP, 1965). In Paragraph 88 of *Publication 26* (ICRP, 1977), the Commission noted that 'flight at high altitude' can increase exposure to natural radiation. In Paragraph 10 of *Publication 39* (ICRP, 1984), 'flying in the present manner' was presented as an example of an existing exposure situation.

(5) The Commission published its first recommendations on protection against exposure to cosmic radiation in *Publication 60* (ICRP, 1991). The Commission recommended that the personnel involved in the operation of commercial jet aircraft be treated as occupationally exposed. As doses are not likely to exceed a pre-defined value because of the limitations of flight duration, the use of dosimeters for individual monitoring was not considered to be necessary. Furthermore, the Commission pointed out that attention should also be paid to groups such as frequent flyers and couriers who fly more often than other passengers. There was no mention of protection of other passengers.

(6) The Commission subsequently clarified its recommendations in *Publication 75* (ICRP, 1997), indicating that because a business traveller could only receive an annual effective dose in the range of 1 mSv (considering approximately 200 h of flying at approximately $5–6 \mu Sv h^{-1}$), the Commission considered that the only group occupationally exposed to elevated levels of cosmic radiation was aircraft crew. The Commission also reiterated that there is no need to consider the use of designated areas in aircraft, that the annual effective doses to aircraft crew should be derived from the flying time and typical effective dose rates for the relevant routes,

and that the control of exposure is mainly ensured by restrictions on flying time and route selection. Recently, a joint publication by the International Commission on Radiation Units and Measurements (ICRU) and ICRP described the cosmic radiation field at aircraft altitudes, and gave reference data for the validation of doses from cosmic radiation to aircraft crew to facilitate international harmonisation of dose assessments for aircraft crew by airlines and their regulators (ICRU, 2010).

(7) This publication supersedes the previous Commission's recommendations related to radiological protection from cosmic radiation in aviation.

1.2. Scope

(8) The Commission has recently published recommendations on controlling exposure to cosmic radiation in space in *Publication 123* (ICRP, 2013). The purpose of the present publication is to update and clarify the recommendations of the Commission on controlling exposure to cosmic radiation in aviation. This publication takes into account the evolution of the general recommendations in *Publication 103* (ICRP, 2007) for the protection of aircraft crew. The publication is intended to enlarge the scope of the discussion beyond aircraft crew by considering the exposure of passengers, notably frequent flyers for personal reasons or professional duties. The publication also addresses the topic of exposure of pregnant women.

1.3. Structure of the publication

(9) Section 2 presents the characteristics of exposure in aviation from cosmic radiation. It provides a brief description of the source and pathways of exposure as well as an overview on solar flares, routine assessment of levels of exposure, and individual and collective dose data. Section 3 describes the ICRP system of radiological protection for cosmic radiation exposure in aviation, including the type of exposure situation, the category of exposure concerned, and the basic principles to be applied. Section 4 provides guidance on implementation of the ICRP system of radiological protection using a graded approach for the various exposed individuals: occasional flyers, frequent flyers, and aircraft crew. A subsection addresses the particular situation of the exposure of pregnant passengers and aircraft crew.

2. CHARACTERISTICS OF EXPOSURE TO COSMIC RADIATION IN AVIATION

2.1. Historical background

(10) In September 1859, R.C. Carrington, an English amateur astronomer, observed a solar flare with a major mass ejection that travelled towards the Earth. Telegraph systems failed rapidly all over Europe and America, and auroras filled the sky as far south as the Caribbean. Today, it is known that solar particle or proton events (SPEs), such as this event in 1859, release relatively high-energy particles that can cause a geomagnetic storm.

(11) In 1912, V. Hess took a historic balloon ride with three ionisation chambers to an altitude of 5300 m. He found higher levels of radiation as he rose, and attributed this to ionising radiation; radiation was four times higher at the peak altitude compared with radiation on the ground. Hess ruled out the Sun as the source of radiation by making several balloon ascents at night and one during a total eclipse. He concluded that 'the results of my observation are best explained by the assumption that a radiation of very great penetrating power enters our atmosphere from above' (Hess, 1912).

(12) In 1925, R.A. Millikan proved the extraterrestrial origin of these radiations, and introduced the terms 'cosmic rays' and 'cosmic radiations'. In the same year, A. Compton proposed that cosmic radiation was primarily charged particles.

(13) Commercial supersonic aircraft were developed during the 1960s: the first flight of the Tupolev-144 prototype was in 1968, while that of the Concorde prototype was in 1969. The high altitude at which supersonic aircraft cruised (approximately 19,000 m) increased concerns regarding the exposure of aircraft crew and passengers to cosmic radiation. To ensure the monitoring of doses, some aircraft crew carried personal dosimeters, and a radiometer was installed in the Concorde. A special dosimeter was also developed for the Tupolev-144's aircraft crew. In the case of a significant increase in radiation level (e.g. $300\,\mu Sv\,h^{-1}$ in the Tupolev-144), the aircraft would descend to a lower altitude. This marked the beginning of routine monitoring of exposure to cosmic radiation in aircraft. Nowadays, the dose from cosmic radiation in aviation is generally estimated using computer codes that have been validated by monitoring results.

2.2. Source and pathways

(14) The Earth is exposed continuously to high-energy particles that come from outside the solar system [galactic cosmic radiation (GCR)] and from the Sun [solar cosmic radiation (SCR)]. In addition, the Earth is exposed occasionally to bursts of energetic particles from the Sun (SPEs). GCR mainly consists of protons (85%) with an energy fluence distribution that extends to more than 10^{20} electron volts (eV). These high-energy particles are a particular characteristic of cosmic radiation, and contribute greatly to the dose. Protons with energies generally below 10^6 eV

constitute 99% of SCR. GCR and SCR are commonly referred to as 'primary cosmic radiation' (UNSCEAR, 2008; ICRU, 2010).

(15) GCR interacts with the atomic constituents of the atmosphere, producing a cascade of interactions and secondary reaction products that contribute to exposure to cosmic radiation (Fig. 2.1). These decrease in intensity with depth in the atmosphere from aircraft altitudes to ground level. The decrease is almost linear between 16 and 8 km of altitude, at $-1.5\,\mu Sv\,h^{-1}\,km^{-1}$ (EC, 2004).

(16) As the particles making up GCR are electrically charged, they can be affected by the magnetic field of the Sun's solar wind (i.e. the plasma of protons and electrons from the solar corona that generates a magnetic field throughout the solar system). The magnetic fields deflect the low-energy GCR that would otherwise enter the Earth's atmosphere. The solar wind varies with the Sun's 11-year solar cycle, and causes variations in the magnetic field. Close to the Earth's orbit, GCR is at a maximum during solar minimum activity, and GCR is at a minimum because of strong solar wind when the Sun's activity is greater, with sunspots, flares, and coronal mass ejections (Fig. 2.2).

(17) Paths of cosmic radiation particles are bent as they cross the magnetic field of the Earth, which acts as a partial shield against charged particles. Near the equator, where the geomagnetic field is nearly parallel to the ground, fewer particles reach

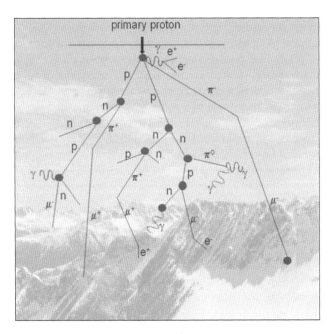

Fig. 2.1. Sketch of cascade of secondary cosmic radiation: μ, muon; e^-, electron; e^+, positron; γ, gamma rays; n, neutron; p, proton; π, pion (picture from W. Rühm).

lower altitudes; the magnetic shielding effect is greater. Near the magnetic poles, where the geomagnetic field is nearly vertical to the ground, the maximum number of primary cosmic radiation particles can reach the atmosphere and generate secondary radiation that penetrates to aviation altitudes. Thus, rates of exposure to cosmic radiation are higher in polar regions, and lower near the equator (Fig. 2.3).

(18) In summary, the cosmic radiation field in aircraft is modulated by altitude, geomagnetic latitude, and solar cycle. At normal aircraft altitudes and at the equator, electrons/positrons and neutrons are the main components in dose, followed by protons. In contrast, at higher latitudes, the dose is mainly from neutrons (Table 2.1). Additionally, at higher altitudes, nuclei heavier than protons (e.g. alpha particles) start to contribute.

2.3. Solar flares

(19) Exceptionally high levels of radiation can occur from solar flares, but only a few (approximately one per year) have significant energies and can be observed by neutron monitors on the ground; these are called 'ground-level enhancements or events' (GLEs). A GLE can cause increases in dose rates at aviation altitudes.

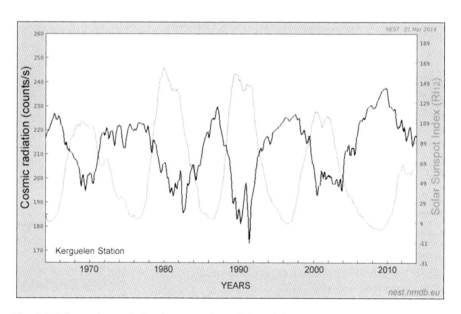

Fig. 2.2. The anti-correlation between the activity of the Sun (expressed as the monthly smoothed number of sunspots; grey curve) and exposure to cosmic radiation (expressed as the monthly average neutron count rates measured at Kerguelen station; black curve) from 1964 to 2014 (IRSN, 2016).

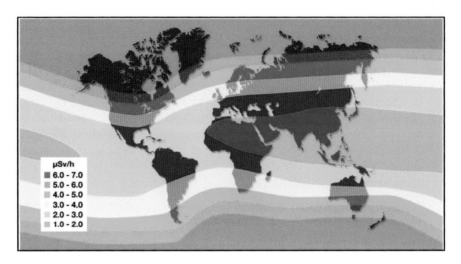

Fig. 2.3. Geomagnetic shielding of cosmic radiation: ambient dose rate by latitude and longitude at an altitude of 11 km in December 2002. Modified from Frasch et al. (2011).

Table 2.1. Contributions to cosmic radiation by its ambient dose equivalent component according to latitude (at altitude of 12,000 m and solar minimum) (EC, 2004).

Component	Equator	Polar latitude
Muons	5%	3%
Electrons/positrons	38%	14%
Neutrons*	37%	64%
Protons	12%	14%
Photons	8%	5%

*The radiation weighting factors for neutrons used in the computation of dose vary as a continuous function of neutron energy (ICRP, 2007). The neutron energy distribution ranges from 10^{-10} to 10^{1} GeV, with maxima at 10^{-3} and 10^{-1} GeV (ICRU, 2010).

Fig. 2.4 shows the daily proton fluence observed by a satellite in October 1989; the solar flare is easily observable.

(20) At present, it is almost impossible to predict the dose of an SPE GLE without large uncertainty (Desmaris, 2006). Calculation of doses to aircraft crew for elevated effective dose rates in the event of an SPE GLE is usually performed retrospectively using results from ground-level neutron monitors or, if available, on-board measurements. The calculated dose rate can be quite substantial, but is characterised by large uncertainties of the order of a factor of 5 or more according to results obtained by EURADOS Working Group 11 (EC, 2004; Beck et al., 2008). According to Lantos and Fuller (2003), 64 GLEs have been observed since 1942, and only

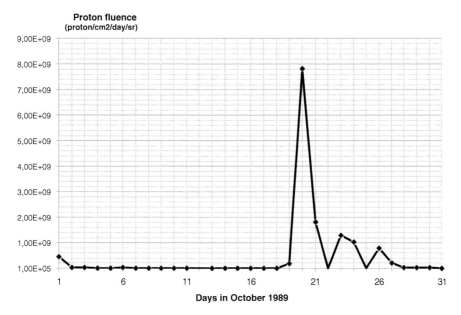

Fig. 2.4. Daily proton fluence between 1 and 31 October 1989 (data obtained from the worldwide web server of the National Atmospheric and Astronautics Administration/ National Geophysical Data Center, USA).

18 of these were associated with a significant likelihood of an increase in the equivalent dose of aircraft crew of more than 30 µSv at 12,000 m. This is comparable to two-thirds of the dose received from GCR during solar maximum for a similar flight. Lantos and Fuller (2003) estimated that only four GLEs could have led to an increase in the dose of more than 1 mSv at 12,000 m. Beck et al. (2008) also concluded that GLEs with a dose higher than a few hundred µSv per flight are rare.

(21) The Commission is aware that concerns have been raised recently about the potential exposure of aircraft crew and passengers to flashes of gamma rays produced in the atmosphere during thunderstorms. This phenomenon, which is not related to cosmic radiation, was first observed by the National Aeronautics and Space Administration in 1991. These flashes, named 'terrestrial gamma-ray flashes', appear to occur at traditional flight altitudes, and last for a few milliseconds with energy up to 20 MeV. The details of their mechanism of production continue to be investigated, but gamma radiation is presumably produced by electrons accelerated by lightning, travelling close to the speed of light, and colliding with atoms in the atmosphere (Dwyer et al., 2012). There is currently no proven/robust procedure to assess the potential exposure of aircraft crew and passengers associated with terrestrial gamma-ray flashes. It is noted that safety procedures require aircraft pilots to alter their course to avoid huge tropical clouds, and not to climb above them (Desmaris, 2016). However, lightning strikes on aircraft occur each year, and

monitoring of all the associated transient events will continue in the coming years. The Commission therefore encourages continued investigation and actions consistent with the optimisation principle as opportunities become reasonable and available.

2.4. Assessment of individual exposure in aircraft

(22) Individual exposure in aircraft can be estimated relatively easily using computer programmes. Indeed, the cosmic radiation field in aircraft is, to a large extent, uniform; for a given flight, the exposure of different individuals is similar (Battistoni et al., 2005). For most computer programmes, the atmosphere is divided into cubes through which the aircraft flies; the mean effective dose rate in a cube depends on altitude, geomagnetic latitude, and solar modulation. The dose when crossing a cube is the product of the dose rate and the time required for the aircraft to cross the cube (Fig. 2.5), which depends on the standard flight profile. The actual flight profile between two airports can differ from the standard flight profile, mainly because of weather conditions, but the impact on the dose is not considered to be significant (Van Dijk, 2003).

(23) Computer codes that evaluate dose rates in aircraft can be validated and consolidated by measurements of ambient dose equivalent rates in the aircraft. For example, in Germany, two passenger aircraft were equipped with ambient dose equivalent rate meters for 4 years in order to validate the calculation programmes used for official dose calculation (Frasch et al., 2014). Details of the determination of ambient dose equivalent rate have been discussed in various consensus standards, such as those by the European Commission (EC, 2004) and the International Organization for Standardization (ISO) Standards ISO 20785 Parts 1–3 (ISO, 2011, 2012, 2013).

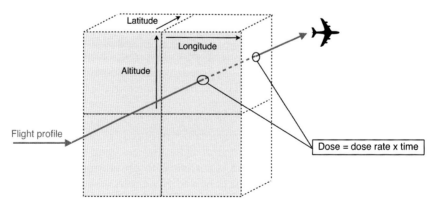

Fig. 2.5. Example of calculation of dose from cosmic radiation used by computer codes (Bottollier-Depois et al., 2007).

(24) EC (2004) has published a compilation of measured and calculated ambient dose equivalent rates covering the time period from 1993 to 2003. These data represent the major basis for the analysis leading to the specification of reference values of ambient dose equivalent given in a joint ICRP and ICRU publication (ICRU, 2010). These reference values can be used to check the conformity of the routine procedure for the assessment of doses to aircraft crew.

(25) Monitoring of occupationally exposed individuals in aircraft has been recommended by ICRP (1997, 2007). As individual doses can be estimated retrospectively, the Commission continues to recommend that the use of validated computer codes be sufficient, instead of using measurement devices (dosimeters and other instruments) to monitor individual exposure in aviation. These codes should fulfil the requirements of relevant authorities. Comparison of such codes has been published recently (EURADOS, 2012).

(26) As an example, the effective doses for three flight routes estimated with a dedicated code can be found in Table 2.2. The value of the dose rate for the trans-equatorial route is the lowest. Other examples of doses for different flight routes can be found in Annex A.

2.5. Exposure of aircraft crew

(27) Data presented by the United Nations Scientific Committee on the Effects of Atomic Radiation (UNSCEAR, 2008) indicate that the range of average annual effective dose for aircraft crew is of the order of a few mSv (1.2–5 mSv depending on the flight routes offered by the airlines in a country), with a maximum value of approximately 6–7 mSv. The average annual effective dose is highly dependent on the average annual flight time, and is of the order of 600 h in European countries and 900 h in the USA. It is of note that these dose estimations, as well as those presented in this publication, are based on *Publication 60* (ICRP, 1991). The Commission is aware that changes in dose calculation introduced in *Publication 103* (ICRP, 2007), such as the radiation weighting factors, will result in a dose that is approximately 30% lower.

(28) A review of the exposure of aircraft crew in Europe (Andresz and Croüail, 2015) indicated that the average annual effective dose varies from 1 mSv for the airline of the Czech Republic to 2.5 mSv for airlines from Finland and Sweden.

Table 2.2. Examples of effective dose calculated for different flight routes (for flights on 15 March 2013).

Type of flight	Total effective dose (μSv)	Average dose rate (μSv h^{-1})
Transatlantic flight: Paris–New York	60	6.8
Transequatorial flight: Colombo–Jakarta	9.7	2
Transpolar flight: Beijing–Chicago	82	6.8

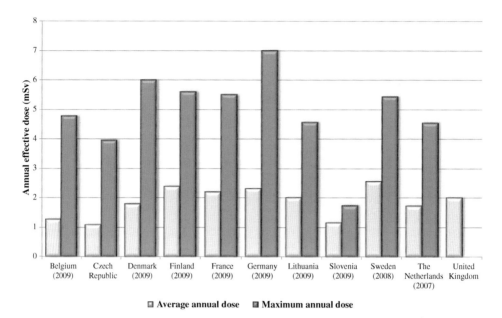

Fig. 2.6. Average and maximum annual effective dose for aircraft crew in European countries (Andresz and Croüail, 2015).

The highest maximum annual effective dose is approximately 6–7 mSv for airlines from Denmark, Germany, and Finland (Fig. 2.6). The average effective dose for aircraft crew in the USA is comparable and was estimated to be 3.1 mSv for 2006 (NCRP, 2009). In Japan, the annual crew doses were evaluated for the year 2007: 1.7 mSv on average and 3.8 mSv at maximum for pilots, and 2.2 mSv on average and 4.2 mSv at maximum for cabin attendants (Yasuda et al., 2011). Apart from exceptional circumstances, aircraft crew receive less than 10 mSv year^{-1}.

(29) Exposure of aircraft crew is also an important component of total occupational exposure. According to UNSCEAR (2008), the total collective annual effective dose of aircraft crew in the world is of the order of 800 man Sv (70–80% of all recorded occupational doses). The collective effective dose per country is largely dependent on the size of the national airline companies and the annual flying time. The collective effective dose can exceed 50 man Sv year^{-1} for certain countries (e.g. 78.5 man Sv for Germany in 2012). Such collective doses represent the main contributor to collective occupational exposure. Table 2.3 represents the collective occupational exposure for aircraft crew in some countries.

(30) The distribution of individual doses received by aircraft crew has the shape of a Gaussian distribution (Fig. 2.7) (in fact, this figure shows the results from the combination of two Gaussian distributions: one for flight deck crew and the other for cabin crew). Such exposure profiles are typical of a population that has a relatively uniform exposure at levels that are sufficiently low that the application of

Table 2.3. Collective dose for aircraft crew (UNSCEAR, 2008).

Country	Monitored individuals	Collective dose (man Sv)
Denmark	3990	6.8
Finland	2520	4.2
Germany	31,000	60.0
Lithuania	160	0.2
The Netherlands	12,500	17.0
UK	40,000	80.0
USA	173,000	531

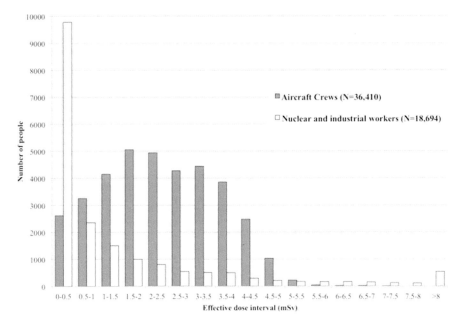

Fig. 2.7. Frequency distribution of annual doses for aircraft crew compared with nuclear and industrial workers in Germany in 2009 (adapted from Frasch et al., 2011).

controls is not warranted. In comparison, the underlying exposure conditions in the nuclear industry are typically much more variable than those in aviation. This fact and the application of the optimisation principle of protection typically result in a much more skewed distribution of doses (e.g. approaching a log-normal distribution).

2.6. Epidemiological studies of aircraft crew

(31) Epidemiological studies of aircraft crew have been conducted over the last 25 years [reviewed by Zeeb et al. (2012)]. The early studies were investigations of pilots from Canada, the UK, and Japan. With regards to cancer, pilots (historically, virtually all pilots were male) showed reduced cancer mortality compared with the general population; this reduction is often observed in occupational cohorts as a healthy worker effect. However, certain specific types of cancers, namely melanoma and brain cancer, seem to be elevated in aircraft crew (Zeeb et al., 2012).

(32) A second generation of investigations in the 1990s included a larger set of European and American studies. As observed previously, cancer mortality of pilots was lower than that of the general population, and some cancers (melanoma and brain cancer) showed 'a very moderate excess risk' (Reynolds et al., 2002). A study also showed a slightly increased risk of cataracts for female cabin crew (females accounted for 80% of the cabin crew, essentially represented by nulliparous women) and 'a very moderate elevation' of breast cancer mortality compared with the general population (Rafnsson, 2005).

(33) UNSCEAR (2006) stated that evidence has been found for consistent excess risk of melanoma, non-melanoma skin cancer, and breast cancer. However, no relationship with the duration of employment was found, and without information on individual radiation dose, it is difficult to correlate the observed excess risks for exposure to ionising radiation or solar ultraviolet light. A recent study found that the incidence of breast cancer is not associated with exposure to cosmic radiation, which may be explained by lower parity and older age at first birth (Schubauer-Berigan et al., 2015).

(34) A study on the mortality of commercial aircraft crew followed 94,000 Europeans and Americans for an average of 22 years (Hammer et al., 2014). This study showed an overall reduction in cancer and cardiovascular mortality compared with the general population. Increased mortality from skin melanoma was observed for flight deck crew, but this was not related directly to occupational exposure and was attributed to light skin and sunbathing. Contrary to other studies, no elevation of breast cancer was found for female aircraft crew, but increased mortality from prostate cancer was observed in male aircraft crew. Generally, mortality from radiation-related cancers was lower than reported in previous analyses. The authors recommended further analysis as aircraft crew are exposed to a number of potential risk factors as well as ionising radiation, including stress, disruption of circadian rhythm, exposure to jet fuel, etc.

(35) In conclusion, the Commission recognises that the available epidemiological data show no clear relationship between the duration of work of aircraft crew, their corresponding doses from cosmic radiation, and an excess risk of radiation-related cancers. Additional evaluation is required that accounts for various potential risk factors as well as ionising radiation.

3. THE ICRP SYSTEM OF PROTECTION FOR PASSENGERS AND AIRCRAFT CREW

(36) The ICRP system of radiological protection of humans is described in *Publication 103* (ICRP, 2007). According to Paragraph 44, it 'applies to all radiation exposures from any source, regardless of its size and origin'. In particular, according to Paragraph 45, the Commission's recommendations cover exposures to both natural and man-made sources.

(37) The philosophy of *Publication 103* (ICRP, 2007) is to recommend a consistent approach for all types of exposure situation, with the central consideration being to keep the optimisation process below appropriate dose restrictions (dose criteria).

3.1. Types of exposure situation and categories of exposure
3.1.1. Types of exposure situation

(38) The Commission defines an exposure situation as a network that begins with a natural or man-made radiation source, the transfer of the radiation or radioactive material through various pathways, and the resulting exposure of individuals [Paragraph 169 in *Publication 103* (ICRP, 2007)]. Protection can be achieved by taking action at the source; at points in the exposure pathways; and occasionally by modifying the location, the time of exposure, and the protection of the exposed individuals. For convenience, the environmental pathway is usually taken to include the link between the source of exposure and the individuals receiving doses.

(39) According to Paragraph 176 of *Publication 103* (ICRP, 2007), the Commission intends its recommendations to be applied to all sources in the following three types of exposure situation, which address all conceivable circumstances.

- Existing exposure situations are exposure situations resulting from sources that already exist when a decision to control the resulting exposure is taken. Characterisation of exposures is a prerequisite for their control.
- Planned exposure situations are situations resulting from the deliberate introduction and operation of sources. Exposures can be anticipated and fully controlled.
- Emergency exposure situations are situations that may occur during the operation of a planned situation in the case of loss of control of the source, or from any unexpected event involving an uncontrolled source. Urgent action is necessary in order to avoid or reduce undesirable exposures.

(40) The Commission views human exposure to cosmic radiation in aviation as an existing exposure situation. The source already exists, and any protection decisions are made in that context to control the exposure. The pathway from the radiation source is outer space, the atmosphere, and the structure and content of the aircraft; and the exposed individuals are the aircraft crew and passengers. Action to control exposures can only be implemented by changing the exposure conditions of the exposed individuals. The Commission considers that GLEs, even major GLEs, are

part of existing exposure situations given their infrequent presence in the flight environment and the resulting small contribution to the exposure of aircraft crew and passengers (see Paragraphs 19 and 20).

(41) The Commission notes that from the standpoint of the protection system, the important factor is the opportunity to optimise protection and take reasonable and effective protective actions for individuals in the particular exposure circumstances. The Commission recognises that many factors affect flight safety, and that aircraft crew are constantly adjusting to the prevailing circumstances. If, at some point in the future, as it becomes reasonable and possible to predict events, improve provision of information to aircraft crew, and take appropriate protective actions, the Commission would expect that authorities and operating managements would respond accordingly as part of the iterative process of optimisation.

3.1.2. Categories of exposure

(42) The Commission distinguishes between three categories of exposure: occupational, public, and medical. Occupational exposure is radiation exposure of workers incurred as a result of their work. However, because of the ubiquity of radiation, the Commission traditionally limits the definition of 'occupational exposures' to radiation exposures incurred at work as a result of situations that can reasonably be regarded as being the responsibility of the operating management. Medical exposure is the exposure of patients in the course of medical diagnosis and treatment. Public exposure encompasses all exposures other than occupational exposures and medical exposures of patients.

(43) In aviation, the population exposed to cosmic radiation includes occasional flyers, frequent flyers for personal reasons or professional duties, and aircraft crew. The Commission maintains its view that the exposure of occasional and frequent flyers is public exposure, and that the exposure of aircraft crew is occupational exposure (ICRP, 1991, 1997, 2007). However, the Commission is now proposing a graded approach for the protection of these three groups, taking into account the level of exposure expected for each group and the responsibilities that need to be considered (Section 4.2).

3.2. Justification of protection strategies

(44) The principle of justification is one of the two fundamental source-related principles that apply to all exposure situations. The recommendation in Paragraph 203 of *Publication 103* (ICRP, 2007) requires, through the principle of justification, that any decision that alters the radiation exposure situation should do more good than harm. The Commission goes on to emphasise that for existing exposure situations, the justification principle is applied in making the decision about whether to take action to reduce exposure and avert further additional exposures. Any decision will always have some disadvantages, and should be justified in the sense that it

should do more good than harm. In these circumstances, as stated in Paragraph 207 of *Publication 103*, the principle of justification is applied in aviation in making the decision about whether to implement a protection strategy against exposure to cosmic radiation.

(45) After characterising the situation, the responsibility for judging the justification usually falls on governments or other national authorities to ensure that an overall benefit results, in the broadest sense to society, and thus not necessarily to each individual. However, input to the justification decision may include many aspects that could be informed by users or other organisations or persons outside of the government or national authority. In this context, radiological protection considerations will serve as input to the broader decision process.

(46) Although possibilities to control exposures in aircraft are limited (Section 4.1), the Commission considers that the implementation of a protection strategy is justified, especially for aircraft crew, given that this is one of the most occupationally exposed populations in terms of both mean individual and collective effective doses (Section 2.5).

3.3. Optimisation of protection

(47) When decisions have been made regarding the justification of implementing a protection strategy, the optimisation of protection becomes the driving principle to select the most effective actions for protecting the exposed individuals.

(48) Optimisation is the second principle that applies to all exposure situations and is central to the ICRP system of radiological protection. It is defined by the Commission as the process to keep the magnitude of individual doses, the number of people exposed, and the likelihood of incurring exposures as low as reasonably achievable below appropriate individual dose criteria, taking into account economic and societal factors. This means that the level of protection should be the best under the prevailing circumstances. In order to avoid serious inequity in individual dose distribution, the Commission recommends the use of individual dose criteria in the optimisation process [Paragraph 226 of *Publication 103* (ICRP, 2007)].

3.3.1. Reference levels

(49) In existing exposure situations, the reference level represents the dose above which it is judged to be inappropriate to plan to allow exposures to occur, for which protective actions should therefore be planned and optimised. Reference levels are guides for selecting protective actions in the optimisation process in order to maintain individual doses as low as reasonably achievable, taking into account economic and societal factors, and thus to prevent and reduce inequities in dose distribution. As such, reference levels are also a benchmark against which protective actions can be judged retrospectively.

(50) For existing exposure situations, the Commission recommends setting reference levels within the 1–20 mSv year^{-1} band, as presented in Table 5 of *Publication 103* (ICRP, 2007). In this band, the sources or pathways can generally be controlled, and individuals receive direct benefits from the activities associated with the exposure situation, but not necessarily from the exposure itself. In aviation, passengers receive direct benefits from flying (i.e. travelling rapidly with comfort and security). Like other situations of occupational exposure to ionising radiation, aircraft crew receive direct benefit from their employment.

(51) For a particular exposure situation, the Commission recommends that the value of the reference level be selected based upon the prevailing circumstances [Paragraph 234 of *Publication 103* (ICRP, 2007)]. This selection should consider the individual dose distribution, with the objective of identifying those exposures that warrant specific attention and contribute meaningfully to the optimisation process. For protection against cosmic radiation in aviation, the Commission recommends that a reference level in the 5–10 mSv year^{-1} range generally be selected.

(52) The selected reference value is not a dose limit, but represents the level of dose below which exposure should be maintained and reduced as low as reasonably achievable, taking into account economic and societal factors. The principle of application of individual dose limits only applies in planned exposure situations [Paragraph 203 of *Publication 103* (ICRP, 2007)]. Nevertheless, some regulatory bodies may decide to introduce occupational dose limits to aircraft crew as a procedure to impose legally binding values.

3.3.2. The optimisation process

(53) In practice, optimisation of protection in existing exposure situations is implemented through a process that involves: (i) assessment of the exposure situation; (ii) identification of the possible protective options to maintain or reduce the exposure to as low as reasonably achievable, taking into account economic and societal factors; (iii) selection and implementation of the most appropriate protective options under the prevailing circumstances; and (iv) regular review of the exposure situation to evaluate if there is a need for corrective actions, or if new opportunities to improve protection have emerged. In this iterative process, the Commission considers that the search for equity in the distribution of individual exposures (i.e. the objective to limit the possibility that some individuals may be subject to much higher exposure than the average in a group exposed under similar circumstances), and the improvement of radiological protection culture are important aspects (ICRP, 2006). When optimising protection, the Commission also recommends 'the need to account for the views and concerns of stakeholders' (ICRP, 2007).

(54) Detailed advice of the Commission on how to apply the optimisation principle in practice has been provided previously (ICRP, 1984, 1991, 2006), and remains valid.

4. IMPLEMENTATION OF THE ICRP SYSTEM OF PROTECTION

4.1. Protective actions

(55) Review of potential protective actions to control exposure in aviation shows that there is little room to manoeuvre. In *Publication 75* (ICRP, 1977), the Commission noted that 'the control of [cosmic radiation] exposure is mainly ensured by restrictions on the flying time and route selection'. Indeed, shielding of the aircraft (fuselage) is not a feasible option. For example, $30\,\mathrm{g\,cm^{-2}}$ shielding is necessary to achieve a 20% reduction in the dose rate at 12,000 m. Even flying time limitation and route selection are difficult actions to implement.

- Flying time limitation. As the dose depends on flight time, work planning of aircraft crew is a means to limit their time in the air. However, limiting the flight time of aircraft crew increases the number of people exposed, and its implementation at large scale may raise societal and economic problems.
- Route selection. It is conceivable to limit exposure by choosing the flight route and acting on altitude and latitude.
  - Altitude. As described in Section 2.2, the Earth's atmospheric layer provides significant shielding from cosmic radiation at typical flight altitudes. Optimisation by flight level is a matter of fine-tuning, taking into account factors such as weather conditions and air traffic, but also cost. For example, it is estimated that reducing flight altitude by 1300 m can reduce dose by 30%. However, this change in altitude increases the risk of accident, and also increases fuel consumption and cost by 5% (Blettner et al., 2014).
  - Latitude. As also described in Section 2.2, the Earth's magnetic field deflects many cosmic radiation particles that would otherwise reach ground level; this effect is most effective at the equator and decreases at higher latitudes. However, optimisation by latitude, particularly re-routing polar flights, increases flight distance, time, and cost.

(56) Regarding exposure during a GLE, it could be envisaged to reduce the altitude of flying aircraft and delay flights that have yet to take off. The implementation of these actions requires the use of sophisticated information systems, which currently remain difficult to develop given technical and organisational considerations. These actions can also disrupt air traffic, which is already tightly scheduled, and increase the potential for accident.

(57) In view of the current options for the control of exposures during flights, the Commission continues to emphasise that the main action to control exposures in aviation is to adjust the flight schedules of the most exposed individuals by consideration of flight time and route selection. For protection in aviation, the Commission now recommends a graded approach according to the level of exposure that individuals are likely to receive, depending on the frequency of their flights.

4.2. Graded approach

(58) Important considerations for protection from cosmic radiation in aviation are the circumstances requiring air travel, the frequency with which an individual may be exposed, and the responsibilities at stake. In this regard, it is important to distinguish between people flying for personal reasons or in the context of their work at the request of their operating management.

(59) For the vast majority of people, the use of air transport is an occasional event, and the dose from cosmic radiation is very low (occasional flyers). The dose becomes higher for a minority of passengers who use aircraft frequently, either privately or in the course of their work (frequent flyers). For this minority of passengers, a simple approach can be to enable these individuals to have the opportunity to assess and understand their exposure. For aircraft crew who generally receive more significant doses, appropriate management of protection is required, based on regular monitoring of all individual doses and modification of the flight roster for those individuals with doses approaching the reference level adopted by the operating management.

4.2.1. Occasional flyers

(60) The Commission is of the view that dose from cosmic radiation received by occasional flyers is sufficiently low that there is no need to warrant the introduction of protection measures.

(61) However, for the sake of transparency and applying the 'right to know' principle, the Commission recommends that general information about cosmic radiation be made available for all passengers, and encourages national authorities, airline companies, consumer unions, and travel agencies to disseminate general information about cosmic radiation associated with aviation. For example, this information could be posted on airlines' websites. These websites could make people aware of the free and validated calculators that estimate flight doses. Annex A gives estimated effective doses for various typical international flight routes.

4.2.2. Frequent flyers for personal reasons or professional duties

(62) Groups of individuals may use aircraft frequently for their personal needs or convenience. Other individuals may fly frequently at the request of their operating management. Most frequent flyers are not exposed to cosmic radiation under the same circumstances as aircraft crew (e.g. in terms of exposure, frequency of flights, and degree of choice). Therefore, the Commission recommends that the exposure of frequent flyers be considered as public exposure (see Paragraph 43), and that individuals exposed be treated in the same way as occasional flyers. The Commission

recommends that general information about cosmic radiation be made available to these individuals.

(63) In addition, the Commission encourages frequent flyers who may be concerned about their exposure to cosmic radiation to assess their personal exposure using freely available dose calculators, in order to be aware of their exposure and adapt their flight frequency if they feel the need.

(64) Among the frequent flyers for professional duties, a very small proportion are exposed under circumstances that result in exposures comparable to exposures of aircraft crew. This may be the case, for example, for couriers transporting documents and materials, or air marshals. The Commission recommends that the exposure of these frequent flyers be managed in a manner similar to the requirements applied for aircraft crew. It is not the intention of the Commission to provide an exhaustive list of the professions at stake, and the decision to consider these frequent flyers as occupationally exposed should be taken on a case-by-case basis according to the prevailing circumstances. This may result in individuals assessing their exposure, and using this information to engage their employer in a dialogue, if appropriate. A decision should result from a process involving all concerned stakeholders.

4.2.3. Aircraft crew

(65) The Commission recommends that airline management inform concerned aircraft crew about radiation and cosmic exposure through ad-hoc educational programmes or training sessions. Information could also be provided to crew at safety meetings, and should be given emphasis in line with other safety issues.

(66) As for any occupationally exposed workers, the Commission recommends that the annual effective dose of each aircraft crew member be assessed. The annual effective dose can be derived from the staff roster and typical effective dose rates using dedicated computer codes. The Commission recommends the occasional use of on-board ambient monitoring, according to the consensus standards, for verification and validation of dose calculations (ICRU, 2010). The Commission does not believe that the contribution of GLEs, in the context of an individual's cumulative exposure, warrants specific monitoring systems such as real-time alert systems. However, the Commission recommends that, whenever reasonably achievable, doses from GLEs be estimated retrospectively and added to the annual exposure of the affected aircraft crew. The Commission also notes that international regulations contain specifications for monitoring equipment for aircraft operating above 15,000 m (ICAO, 2010).

(67) The Commission also recommends that aircraft crew doses be recorded, and that annual and cumulative individual doses be made available on request from the individual. To facilitate potential epidemiological studies, this information should be kept for a reasonable period of time that is, at a minimum, comparable with the expected lifetime of the individuals (ICRP, 1997).

Table 4.1. Recommendations of the Commission for individuals exposed to cosmic radiation in aviation.

	Exposed individuals	Recommendations	Categories of exposure
Reference level to be selected in the 5–10 mSv year^{-1} range	Occasional flyers	• General information	Public
	Frequent flyers	• General information • Self-assessment of doses • Individual initiative to adjust flight frequency as appropriate	Public*
	Aircraft crew	• Individual information • Assessment of individual doses • Recording of individual doses • No specific additional medical surveillance • Adjustment of flight roster as appropriate	Occupational

*Some groups of frequent flyers may be managed in a manner similar to those occupationally exposed, decided on a case-by-case basis according to the prevailing circumstances.

(68) Aircraft crew routinely undergo medical examinations for reasons other than radiation safety. The Commission considers that exposure to cosmic radiation does not require specific additional medical examinations. Generally, routine medical examinations represent an opportunity to engage a dialogue between a worker and a physician on the topic of exposure to cosmic radiation.

(69) When judged appropriate and in order to respect the selected dose reference level, the operating management may adjust the roster of the concerned individual (frequency and/or destination).

4.2.4. Summary

(70) Table 4.1 lists the recommendations of the Commission regarding the exposure of individuals to cosmic radiation.

4.3. Protection of embryo and fetus

(71) In *Publication 82* (ICRP, 1999), the Commission concluded that prenatal exposure in the case of an existing exposure situation does not require protective

actions, other than those for the general population. The Commission does not therefore believe that actions to adjust flight rosters of pregnant women will be necessary. Women who fly frequently and may be or expect to be pregnant should be provided with sufficient information to make informed judgements regarding the flight rosters and any adjustment they may wish to consider.

(72) Regarding occupationally exposed aircraft crew, it is the Commission's recommendation that the methods of protection at work for pregnant women provide a level of protection of the embryo/fetus from ionising radiation that is broadly similar to that provided for members of the public. In Paragraph 186 of *Publication 103* (ICRP, 2007), the Commission recommended that 'Once an employer has been notified of a pregnancy, additional protection of the embryo/fetus should be considered. The working conditions of a pregnant worker, after declaration of pregnancy, should be such as to ensure that the additional dose to the embryo/fetus would not exceed about 1 mSv during the remainder of the pregnancy.'

(73) Generally, female workers are encouraged to report their pregnancy to their employer as soon as possible. In some countries, the decision is a voluntary matter for the individuals. Irrespective of these differences, pregnant crew may receive more than 1 mSv before declaring the pregnancy. To encourage the timely declaration of pregnancy, the Commission recommends that female aircraft crew and frequent flyers be informed about the risks for the embryo/fetus from exposure to cosmic radiation. After the declaration, provision should be made during the remainder of the pregnancy.

4.4. Information dissemination to the general public and stakeholder engagement

(74) Aside from experienced scientists, experts, and professionals trained in radiological protection, citizens are usually not well informed about ionising radiation and their potential health effects. On the matter of exposure to cosmic radiation, apart from most aircraft crew, few people among the general public are aware of this exposure, although they are constantly exposed to cosmic radiation in everyday life on the ground, and at an elevated level when travelling in aircraft. However, in recent years, there has been growing information on cosmic phenomena, particularly solar flares, disseminated by space and weather organisations, and relayed by the media, occasionally giving rise to airline alerts. This information has awakened the attention of some passengers to cosmic radiation, but also raised questions and sometimes concerns among frequent flyers and aircraft crew about the risks associated with exposure to cosmic radiation.

(75) In accordance with the 'right to know' principle, which states that people have the right to be informed about the potential risks that they may be exposed to in their daily life, and the underlying ethical values of autonomy, justice, and prudence, the Commission encourages national authorities, airline companies, consumer unions, and travel agencies to disseminate general information about cosmic radiation associated with aviation. This information must be easily accessible and should present

the origins of cosmic radiation; the influence of altitude, latitude, and solar cycle; and indicate typical doses associated with a set of traditional flight routes and the potential of receiving unexpected exposure in the case of a rare but intense GLE.

(76) As mentioned in Sections 2.4 and 4.2, several easy-to-use tools have been made available on the Internet in recent years. These tools allow dose calculations to be made for all flights.

(77) The Commission recommends that the general information on cosmic radiation be such that the messages are accurate, informative, and responsive to the nature of the concerns and challenges in terms of radiological protection according to the situation. The Commission suggests that cosmic radiation should be viewed in proportion with other risks or considerations, to foster a more inclusive view of all risks so that individuals can make informed decisions.

(78) From this perspective, comparison with other exposure situations to natural and man-made radiation sources may be useful (e.g. a flight from London to New York gives the same effective dose as spending 10 days on holiday in a high mountain region), and should be made accessible as part of the general information on cosmic radiation. However, such comparisons must be undertaken with care, because the perception and tolerability of risk depend largely on the characteristics of the situation, particularly the degree to which the situation is taken to be a personal decision, and the benefit for the individuals of the activities that lead to the exposures.

(79) The Commission considers that, regarding protection against cosmic radiation in aviation, passengers who are not occupationally exposed must remain accountable for their choices, but that these choices should be made knowingly based on relevant information without bias. The decision by individuals to reduce the frequency of their flights will be based on personal considerations, for which the risk of exposure to cosmic radiation is only one element among many others. Finally, it is up to the individual taking the risk to judge its tolerability based on accurate information, and to make decisions for their own protection.

5. CONCLUSIONS

(80) The Earth is bombarded continuously by particles from deep space and the Sun. The atmosphere and the Earth's geomagnetic field provide sufficient shielding that exposure at ground level is not of particular concern, but exposure to cosmic radiation increases with altitude. This existing exposure situation is experienced by millions of travellers: passengers for personal reasons or on request of their operating management, and aircraft crew who are among the most highly exposed occupational populations.

(81) The Commission notes that occasional flights only contribute a very small increment of the dose received annually due to natural background radiation at ground level, and does not warrant the introduction of protection measures. It is recognised that some passengers may, for personal and very different reasons, be concerned about exposure to cosmic radiation. The Commission thus recommends the dissemination of relevant information to allow them to make informed decisions.

(82) For frequent flyers for personal reasons or professional duties, the Commission also recommends the dissemination of relevant information, and moreover that individuals avail themselves of opportunities for self-assessment of their exposure in order to consider adjustment of flight frequency as appropriate. For particular groups of frequent flyers for professional duties who accumulate flight durations similar to those of aircraft crew, the Commission recommends that they engage in discussions with their organisations in order to manage their exposure, with requirements similar to those for aircraft crew.

(83) For the protection of aircraft crew, the Commission maintains its previous recommendations, and introduces the use of a reference level to be selected by operating managements. Values in the $5–10\,\text{mSv year}^{-1}$ range are generally appropriate. The specific level selected should take into account the prevailing circumstances, so that the value can contribute meaningfully to the optimisation process. The available options to reduce exposures from cosmic radiation are very limited. The most effective option is the adjustment of flight rosters when doses are approaching the selected reference level.

(84) With the above recommendations, the Commission expects to keep doses of the most exposed individuals – aircraft crew and some frequent flyers – as low as reasonably achievable below the selected reference levels. The Commission also anticipates that by raising general awareness about exposure to cosmic radiation in aviation, a more informed dialogue among stakeholders can take place. All involved stakeholders – occasional flyers, frequent flyers, and aircraft crew – are encouraged to make informed decisions with regard to the exposures associated with flying, and also to consider all the benefits they receive from air travel.

REFERENCES

Andresz, S., Croüail, P., 2015. Results of the EAN request on the radiological protection of aircrew. European ALARA Newsletter n°36. Available at: www.eu-alara.net (last accessed 14 May 2016).

Battistoni, G., Ferrari, M., Pelliccioni, M., Villari, R., 2005. Evaluation of the dose to aircrew members taking into consideration aircraft structure. Adv. Space Res. 36, 1645–1652.

Beck, P., Bartlett, D.T., Bilski, P., et al., 2008. Validation of modelling the radiation exposure due to solar particle events at aircraft altitudes. Radiat. Prot. Dosim. 131, 51–58.

Blettner, M., Boehm, T., Bottollier-Depois, J-F., et al., 2014a. Strahlenexposition beim Fliegen – Ein Fall für den Strahlenschutz, Strahlenschutz Praxis, Heft 2, 3–30. TÜV Media Gmbh, Köln.

Bottollier-Depois, J.F., Blanchard, P., Clairand, I., et al., 2007. An operational approach for aircraft crew dosimetry: the SIEVERT system. Radiat. Prot. Dosim. 125, 421–424.

Desmaris, G., 2006. Is space weather forecast worthwhile for an airline in terms of radiation protection? Proceedings of the 54th International Congress of the International Academy of Aviation and Space Medicine, 2006, Bangalore, India.

Desmaris, G., 2016. Cosmic radiation in aviation: radiological protection of Air France aircraft crew. Ann. ICRP 45(1S), 64–74.

Dwyer, J., Smith, D., Cummer, S., 2012. High energy atmospheric physics: terrestrial gamma-ray flashes and related phenomena. Space Sci. Rev. 133, 133–196.

EC, 2004. Radiation Protection 140, Cosmic Radiation Exposure of Aircraft Crew – Compilation of Measured and Calculated Data. European Radiation Dosimetry Group (EURADOS), Braunschweig.

EURADOS, 2012. EURADOS Report 2012–03. Comparison of Codes Assessing Radiation Exposure of Aircraft Crew due to Galactic Cosmic Radiation. European Radiation Dosimetry Group, Braunschweig. Available at: http://www.eurados.org/~/media/Files/Eurados/documents/EURADOS_Report_201203.pdf (last accessed 14 May 2016).

Frasch, G., Kammerer, L., Karofsky, R., Schlosser, A., Spiesl, J., Stegemann, R., 2011. Die berufliche Strahlenexposition des fliegenden Personals in Deutschland 2004 – 2009. BfS-SG-15/11. Bundesamt für Strahelneschutz, Salzgitter, p. 42. Available at: https://doris.bfs.de/jspui/bitstream/urn:nbn:de:0221-201108016029/3/Bf_2011_BfS-SG-15-11-ExpositionFlugPersonal.pdf (last accessed 14 May 2016).

Frasch, G., Kammerer, L., Karofsky, R., Schlosser, A., Stegemann, R., 2014. Radiation exposure of German aircraft crews under the impact of solar cycle 23 and airline business factors. Health Phys. 107, 542–554.

Hammer, G.P., Auvinen, A., De Stravola, B.L., et al., 2014. Mortality from cancer and other causes in commercial airlines crews: a joint analysis of cohorts from 10 countries. Occup. Environ. Med. 71, 313–322.

Hess, V.F., 1912. Über Beobachtungen der durchdringenden Strahlung bei sieben Freiballonfahrten. Physikalische Zeitschrift 13, 1084–1091.

ICAO, 2010. Annex 6, Operation of Aircraft, Part I, International Commercial Air Transport – Aeroplanes, ninth edition. International Civil Aviation Organization, Montreal.

ICAO, 2015. Air Navigation Report, International Civil Aviation Organization, 2015 Edition, Montreal.

ICRP, 1965. Recommendations of the International Commission on Radiological Protection. ICRP Publication 9. Pergamon Press, Oxford.

ICRP, 1977. Recommendations of the ICRP. ICRP Publication 26. Ann. ICRP 1(3).

ICRP, 1984. Principles for limiting exposure of the public to natural sources of radiation. ICRP Publication 39. Ann. ICRP 14(1).

ICRP, 1991. Recommendations of the International Commission on Radiological Protection. ICRP Publication 60. Ann. ICRP 21(1–3).

ICRP, 1997. General principles for the radiation protection of workers. ICRP Publication 75. Ann. ICRP 27(1).

ICRP, 1999. Protection of the public in situations of prolonged radiation exposure. ICRP Publication 82. Ann. ICRP 29(1/2).

ICRP, 2006. The optimisation of radiological protection: broadening the process. ICRP Publication 101b. Ann. ICRP 36(3).

ICRP, 2007. The 2007 Recommendations of the International Commission on Radiological Protection. ICRP Publication 103. Ann. ICRP 37(2–4).

ICRP, 2013. Assessment of radiation exposure of astronauts in space. ICRP Publication 123. Ann. ICRP 42(4).

ICRP, 2014. Radiological protection in security screening. ICRP Publication 125. Ann. ICRP 43(2).

ICRU, 2010. Reference data for the validation of doses from cosmic-radiation exposure of aircraft crew. Report 84. J. ICRU 10(2).

IRSN, 2016. SIEVERT version 2.2.4. Fontenay-aux-Roses, France. Available at: https://www.sievert-system.org/?locale=en#Rayonnement (last accessed 14 May 2016).

ISO, 2011. ISO 20785. Dosimetry for Exposures to Cosmic Radiation in Civilian Aircraft – Part 2: Characterization of Instrument Response. International Organization for Standardization, Geneva.

ISO, 2012. ISO 20785. Dosimetry for Exposures to Cosmic Radiation in Civilian Aircraft – Part 1: Conceptual Basis for Measurements. International Organization for Standardization, Geneva.

ISO, 2013. ISO 20785. Dosimetry for Exposures to Cosmic Radiation in Civilian Aircraft – Part 3: Measurements at Aviation Altitude. International Organization for Standardization, Geneva.

Lantos, P., Fuller, N., 2003. History of the solar particle event radiation doses on-board aeroplanes using semi-empirical model and Concorde measurements. Radiat. Prot. Dosim. 104, 199–210.

NCRP, 2009. Ionising Radiation Exposure of the Population of the United States. NCRP Report 160. National Council on Radiation Protection and Measurements, Bethesda, MD.

Rafnsson, V., 2005. Cosmic radiation increases the risk of nuclear cataract in airline pilots. Arch. Ophthalmol. 123, 1102–1105.

Reynolds, P., Cone, J., Layefsky, M., et al., 2002. Cancer incidence in Californian flight attendants. Cancer Causes Control. 13, 317–324.

Schubauer-Berigan, M.K., Anderson, J.L., Hein, M.J., et al., 2015. Breast cancer incidence in a cohort of U.S. flight attendants. Am. J. Ind. Med. 58, 252–266.

The New York Times, 1924. Lindbergh Does It! To Paris in 33 1/2 Hours; Flies 1,000 Miles Through Snow and Sleet; Cheering French Carry Him Off Field. 21 May 1924. The New York Times, New York. Available at: http://www.nytimes.com/learning/general/onthis day/big/0521.html (last accessed 14 May 2016).

UNSCEAR 2006. Effects of Ionizing Radiation, Report to the General Assembly, Volume 1, Annex A: Epidemiological Studies of Radiation and Cancer. United Nations, New York.

UNSCEAR, 2008. Sources and Effects of Ionizing Radiation, Report to the General Assembly with Scientific Annexes, Volume I, Annex B: Exposures from Natural Radiation Source. United Nations, New York.

Van Dijk, J.W., 2003. Dose assessment of aircraft crew in the Netherlands. Radiat. Prot. Dosim. 106, 25–31.

Yasuda, H., Sato, T., Yonehara, H., et al., 2011. Management of cosmic radiation exposure for aircrew in Japan. Radiat. Prot. Dosim. 146, 123–125.

Zeeb, H., Hammer, G.P., Blettner, M., 2012. Epidemiological investigations of aircrew: an occupational group with low-level cosmic radiation exposure. J. Radiol. Prot. 32, 15–19.

ANNEX A. COSMIC RADIATION EXPOSURE ASSOCIATED WITH SELECTED FLIGHT ROUTES

Table A.1. Cosmic radiation exposure associated with selected flight routes.

	Abu Dhabi (Emirates)	Johannesburg	Kuala Lumpur	Lima	London	Mexico (city)	Moscow	New York (city)	Rio de Janeiro (city)	Tokyo	San Francisco	Sydney
Abu Dhabi (Emirates)		0.016	0.012	0.052	0.04	0.03	0.012	0.077	0.031	0.07	0.109	0.058
Johannesburg	0.016		0.049	0.048	0.015	0.036	0.058	0.005	0.015	0.016	0.024	0.028
Kuala Lumpur	0.012	0.049		0.029	0.072	0.016	0.019	0.124	0.031	0.012	0.057	0.042
Lima	0.052	0.048	0.029		0.052	0.013	0.065	0.019	0.014	0.058	0.022	0.072
London	0.04	0.015	0.072	0.052		0.079	0.058	0.004	0.011	0.08	0.08	0.075
Mexico (city)	0.03	0.036	0.016	0.013	0.079		0.032	0.045	0.023	0.062	0.005	0.078
Moscow	0.012	0.058	0.019	0.065	0.058	0.032		0.064	0.02	0.014	0.134	0.039
New York (city)	0.077	0.005	0.124	0.019	0.004	0.045	0.064		0.025	0.095	0.03	0.058
Rio de Janeiro (city)	0.031	0.015	0.031	0.014	0.011	0.023	0.02	0.025		0.126	0.02	0.102
Tokyo	0.07	0.016	0.012	0.058	0.08	0.062	0.014	0.095	0.126		0.043	0.07
San Francisco	0.109	0.024	0.057	0.022	0.08	0.005	0.134	0.03	0.02	0.043		0.06
Sydney	0.058	0.028	0.042	0.072	0.075	0.078	0.039	0.058	0.102	0.07	0.06	

Effective doses (in mSv) calculated for March 2016 using the SIEVERT software (http://www.sievert-system.org/index.html).